Lee Has Yellow Eyes
Understanding Sickle Cell

Latoya Harris
Illustrated Latoya Harris Reshaud Kidd

Foreword

I was glad when I heard my mom (La'Toya Harris-Kidd) said she was done with the book. I knew it was going to help bring much needed attention to sickle cell. I have had sickle cell all my life and although it's not the easiest illness to live with you learn to be as strong as you have to be to get through the hard times the invisible disease brings. I have been through so much in the past three years because of sickle cell. I recently had a stroke and temporarily lost my ability to speak.

I hope the book helps other families that are going through the hard times and it shines some light on some questions that you readers may have. I want others to just simply be aware of the things that the invisible disease is capable of doing and help find a cure. I'm not looking for sympathy or pity, I only want awareness and recognition to what we go through with sickle cell anemia.

I write this brief shout out to my mom La'Toya Harris-Kidd for writing this amazing book based on my life with sickle cell. I feel this book will be a great book for both children and adults that are interested in learning how to cope with sickle cell. As for me, I feel so blessed and honored to be a part of such a great and positive project and I am looking forward to all the great reactions to this book. We're breaking down barriers MOM!!!!!

Reshaud Kidd #SICKLECELLKIDD

PREFACE

Lee is a character I created based off of my son who has sickle cell anemia. I remember getting the call from his doctor when he was three days old telling me that he had a blood disorder called sickle cell disease. I was a single young mother scared that I did something to cause this and he had it because of something that I did. Left to handle majority of the responsibility I did what I had to do to take care of my family. Growing up in what most call the hood I had limited outlets and many ways to make a quick dollar which was appealing for a struggling mother. I thought I was being punished and so I lived with that inside for a long time.

The book is about *Lee* a young boy who gets asked all the time why his eyes are yellow and what sickle cell is. He started to tell people things his doctor and nurses would tell him and found many did not have a clue to what it was like. So *Lee* became my son's voice, once he had something to express through he did not feel so on the spot because his character sort of took over in his imagination. Throughout my sons illness our family had gone through a lot of ups and downs because of financial situations things were often a stretch to make.

I wrote the book sort of on an accident because I always expressed myself through writing and drawing. Being a young mom I felt the need to know as much as I could to prove that I could handle the care of my family. Keeping our struggles to myself because I knew everyone had their own issues left me on my own many times. Once my son reached eighteen I felt accomplished and I felt that I had done the main part of my job and then my worst nightmare happened. He had a stroke his senior year of high school, I was devastated and alone but my close friends came and through social media I did receive prayers along with encouraging comments. So with that and a few more bumps in the road I compiled all that I had written and tailored my character around some of the events.

The purpose of the book is to inform those who are not aware of sickle cell anemia and give them an inside look from the child and family's point of view. I want to give ways of coping with the pain, encourage art therapy in rehabilitation, and advocate for sickle cell. Let everyone know that this is a life threatening illness that needs a cure and explain what sickle cell is, what happens during a crisis and what to do after you get out of the hospital. My goal is to bring awareness to sickle cell anemia and help them live a productive life until all the research pays off with a cure.

It took me three years to write this book but I have notes, journals, and records that goes back twenty years. This book is for both children and adults which makes it a tool for teaching in a modern form. My son had to learn how to talk again and I used music, art, along with his medical rehab combining the arts with the facts kept it approachable in an honest open form of expression. I often look at art, literature, music, and technology as branches through generation's trees that are rooted deep all which are ways we can find some common ground.

I am very proud of my work although I am always my worst critic I wrote it a hundred times but when I closed my eyes I had a vision. I could actually see all of my ideas in my head so I drew them, I poured all of my experiences as a mother and I fulfilled a dream of becoming not only an author, illustrator, but most of all an advocate for a cause that I hold so close to my heart.

I would like to thank my first husband and friend Freddie Kidd for always being there for me regardless of the situation you're always real, encourage me and will forever have a special place in my heart. I want to thank my sons Freddie III, Reshaud, and Cameron and my daughters Cheneah and Lyric for understanding me and allowing me to grow as I became the mom you all deserve. I would also like to thank my grandma's Clarice and Julia for giving me all the strength, wisdom, and making me tough. I can't forget my mom, pops and my dad for being the best parents they could be. They did what they could for me, I didn't turn out too bad and thanks to all my siblings for having my back and letting me practice being a mom on you.

INTRO

Have you ever known a child who required special care sometimes, or maybe all of the time? All children need to be cared for in an attentive way but some children require a little more attention by the adults in their life. They may require special equipment to get around like a wheelchair, medication, a lot of doctor appointments, and sometimes they might need to stay home or go to the hospital and stay a few days. This is a story about one of those children and his name is Lee. What makes him require special attention at times is he was born with Sickle cell disease which is not contagious, it is a genetic disorder? When you hear the word genetic it means inherited through genes from your parents and their parents, grandparents and so on.

Lee is going to describe how sickle cell affects his life he will go over what sickle cell disease is, a pain crisis and what happens when he has one. The care for a person with an illness requires specific routines for daily living which is handled by your parents but when you have an illness you have to learn how to take care of yourself as well. Lee will walk you through several situations that come along with having sickle cell. Understanding the illness, how it affects the quality of not only his life but his family's as well. This is his family's story of living with sickle cell and how to cope in a positive way.

To the human eye he was just like any little brown boy in the neighborhood running down the street waving a dollar bill in one hand, as he ran towards the song of the ice cream truck screaming, "Stttooooopp!!". Like any boy he was easily distracted by his short attention span, video games, Pokemon, and fighting over the remote. He raced back in the house with ice cream dripping down his arm to reclaim his sunk in cushion so he could watch his favorite show on cartoon network. He was a little out of breath because he had to race not only reclaim his favorite spot on the couch but the remote to the TV. That way he can watch his favorite shows then pass it on to the sibling of his choice. That is unless his big brother pull rank and wrestle him for the remote but by then Lee knew he would have already watched two shows because he gets home before his thirteen year old big brother Angel.

Having a big brother and younger sister often left Lee stuck in the middle and basically the tiebreaker to every vote that took place at 429 Bluff Cove. His family was very important to him just like any eleven year old boy. Lee loved when he gets the chance to go with his dad to work because he fixed motorcycles for the best bike maker in America Harley Davidson. His mom was a beautician and she had her own hair salon that is our second home. We all say that because my mom is always there if she is not at home with us. I have a little eight year old sister we call her Minnie because she looks like a little version of mom (she acts like her too…sometimes she was very bossy). At the end of the day my mom is home preparing dinner, inspecting chores and homework at the same time while she cleans up the house. She is like a superhero when it comes to our family have you ever looked in the refrigerator at least five times and didn't see anything to eat then your mom comes home open it up and make an entire meal. That is magic making something out of nothing, putting the right pieces together makes the puzzle complete even if the pieces aren't perfect they all have their special place.

If you look at most families we all have our way of living and getting through life together but the key is communicating and understanding. Raising an African-American or any other minority can be a challenge when you face neighborhoods that are not so fortunate. Now a parent with a child who has a serious long-term medical condition is quite often overwhelmed with the demands of the illness. Many careers fail due to your child being sick and out of school frequently it will cause you to be absent from work. If you are not with your company longer than one year you have limited options but if you have been employed a year or longer you would qualify for FMLA which is the Family Medical Leave Act (check with your human resources department for details). A parent will always choose their child first but you also have to provide for your family so choosing a career and finding support to help with babysitting, running errands, so that you can get that promotion and do your job well is crucial.

There are community groups, family, friends that can help when you as a parent feel the burden weighing heavy or simply just feeling alone. As a mom hearing all of the medical issues your child has caused by a trait inherited from you can be a huge part of the burden and add to any guilt you feel, that's when you need to talk to someone like a therapist if a friend is not enough. Not knowing by negligence only highlights the fact that we need to have genetic counseling before deciding to have children and that needs to be done at an early age because although it is not encouraged but people have been having children as teens for a long time. That way we would be aware of what traits we can pass on and what genes we were born with.

Overall the family will be the foundation of support for the simple fact that when we are hurt we reach out to them first and if there is a serious illness going on you always reach out to who is closest to you. If not for comfort for education so you can learn about other family members who have had the same illness as well as different resources. Knowledge is important but if we don't use it then it is worth anything. There will be a time when you have to begin to talk to your child and let them know how important it is to tell you when they are hurting. Reassuring them that you will use every way possible way to ease the pain, giving them hugs through the many doctor visits will be a lifelong journey but knowing they can count on you will ease the edge off the pain.

Minimizing the facts, living in denial can only hurt that baby you carried to term and to protect your child you cannot ignore the truth there is no running from this in the end it is up to you to take care of your child until that child can take care of themself.

You can show your child through art what blood cells are, how sickle cells look to make it relatable. Explain why it is important for your child to drink a lot of water in all weather, any extreme weather temperature can be hard for your child. They should know this for when they spend the night or go on field trips that staying warm in cold and cool in heat is vital for their health. Cold and high altitudes is not good for someone with sickle cell knowing these simple things will help your child prevent many health issues. Letting your child know that you will always will be there is crucial for them growing up and will give them confidence to one day be able to handle their own care for the most part. Keeping any child grounded is important and holding them accountable for their actions is important even if they have an illness they must know that they are just like everyone else they just have to learn their own limitations. Having siblings can be a challenge but also gives the balance if you focus. I never limit my expectations of Lee although he has boundaries he was taught that even on his bad day he is still good at what he puts his mind and name to #SICKLECELLKIDD.

FACT: Hemoglobin is a protein that carries oxygen to all parts of the body. Having anemia comes from your blood not carrying enough oxygen to the rest of your body. Lee was born with a blood disorder called "Sickle Cell Anemia" this is a disease which causes your body to produce abnormally shaped red blood cells that is shaped like a crescent or a sickle which causes the cells to clog in vessels. This can lead to severe pain and damage to tissue. Blood cells shaped like this they do not last as long as the normal round shaped blood cells and this is what steers towards anemia.

Contents

1

Who is Lee

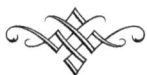

Standing in the mirror early in the morning a boy looked at his reflection and what stood out to him, as he gazed in the mirror was the whites of his eyes were yellow today, again. He sighed, as he continued with his normal routine of brushing his teeth and washing his face.

My name is Lee, and I'm going to tell you about me and invite you into my world. Having Sickle Cell Disease has given me a great imagination, especially when I am in the hospital for a while. If I get admitted to the hospital for a pain episode I'm not able to go outside for a few days and that seems like an eternity. I love the fresh air and the wind as it blows on my skin. So while I heal I bring what is outside to me by using my imagination when my family and friends visit and tell me about their day I can only put myself in their shoes and see what they describe as if I was standing right there with them.

Many of you may have a pet and because I have allergies my parents are hesitant because I may be allergic and they are not too excited about the idea of a cat or dog so I keeps getting fish. I am working on wearing them down by asking for a dog every birthday, holiday and basically every chance I get. So far the answer is still "No" because the dog may be too much responsibility for me, right now. I doubt that I am the only one who has or had an imaginary friend. I have had mines my whole life and sometimes I wish it will go away when it causes trouble. It can be a problem because I am the only one that can see and feel it. There are times I did things and I blamed it on my imaginary friend SS he causes me a lot of trouble especially the times I can't explain when blame it when something goes wrong. I had to learn to I should not use it as an excuse not to take care of my responsibilities like chores or homework because I would not be able to have fun and when I am really sick they might not believe me. I am learning about my own illness by asking questions it will be me who would has to live with sickle cell for the rest of my life unless they find a cure other than my parents having another child to do a bone marrow transplant which is the only known cure so far.

If you have not noticed my imaginary friend is my illness "sickle cell" this is because often when people look at me they are not able to tell that I have an illness and this way I get used to it always being around. That is why I call it my pet because we are in this together. My pet SS, yeah I know what you're thinking that is a strange name for a pet but that is his name because he looks like a sickle cell with his crescent shape and the type I have is SS. There are a few types of sickle cell like there are a few types of diabetes (which is another illness). My SS is the most common type caused by inheriting one gene from each parent. It is also possible to inherit sickle cell from only one parent with the sickle cell trait if the other parent has another form of anemia like hemoglobin C, D, E, or thalassemia.

When I get sick I have pain episodes which will happen often, organ and tissue damage is another result of my illness. Our organ the spleen is the bodies filter that removes red blood cells that are damaged and is very important for the immune system creating the white blood cells that fight infection so it is often checked to see if it is enlarged. The anemia can range from moderate to severe so during my routine check-ups I have to go to the lab and get my blood drawn. They put it in a few different tubes with different colors. Going to the doctor to see my hematology team they are a group of doctors who treat blood disorders.

To keep it between us he is a sickle cell and when I go into my world he and I go on many adventures on our journey back to health.

You see I had to become friends with what many people might say is my enemy. At first I use to get mad at it and wonder why did I get stuck with it then I had a dream one night in the hospital after my mom told me that I was the strongest little guy that she knew and I gave her strength. She said I was her hero and we could cry and be sad or we can fight together while we all get through this as a family and I was not alone. I made peace with my enemy in my dream that night and we decided to fight together. Since we are bonded together through life I accepted what I had and we became friends.

FACT: Those with sickle cell anemia may develop jaundice (pronounced: jon-dis), a condition that results from the high rate of red blood cell breakdown. Jaundice can cause the whites of a person's eyes to develop a yellowish tint. Children that have sickle cell disease break down more red blood cells so they have more amounts of bilirubin, which is a byproduct of red blood cells.

He walked over to the medicine cabinet and as he opened its door he heard his mother yell from the kitchen, "make sure you take your medicine", rolling his eyes he replied, "I'm doing that right now". He had to take a folic acid (folate) tablet every day this helps me make new red blood cells. By having an increased risk for infection I took daily penicillin until I was six years old my mom got the flavored liquid so I never noticed. When I take my medicine everyday it is like feeding my pet, making sure it has the right nutrients to be healthy. I have to do this every day so that I prevent any complications it is like when you walk your dog you have to put it on a leash to prevent him from getting out of control.

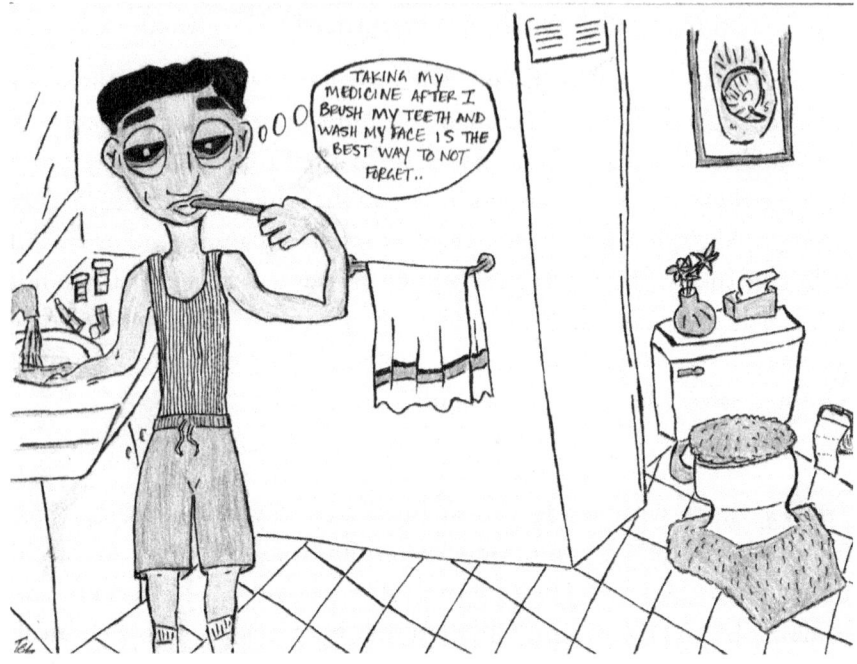

Lee's mom called out to him, "Also, can you come here so I can take your temperature". Lee responded by yelling out, "okay" closing the bathroom door behind him as he ran down the stairs.

FACT: Folic acid is a "B" vitamin, and it helps his body make new cells and helps the type of anemia he was born with. This is Sickle Cell Anemia or disease this affects hemoglobin in red blood cells.

His mom does this just about every morning, pulls out the thermometer and checks to see if I has a fever. She says it is a preventative measure she takes and it helps her know how my insides are feeling. With Sickle Cell it helps to be cautious and do things like get a flu shot, cover your mouth, dress according to the weather outside so my mom likes to put layers of clothes on me so if it is hot I can pull off my long sleeve and coat and have a short sleeve on. She says with Sickle Cell it is always good to be careful and try to stay a step ahead of an illness which keeps me two steps away from a pain crisis, my mom says.

Most of us can look back at childhood and remember a few experiences that will stay in our memories forever. This was when we had no worries, we played for hours with our favorite toys. We would eat whatever we was placed on the dinner table and snacked on junk food all day. When a person who does not have a serious illness catches a common cold it sucks but when you have sickle cell it can really be bad and lead to a pain crisis if not properly diagnosed and treated because it is harder for them to fight infections. Any other time someone catches a cold you can treat it with basic over the counter remedies and maybe a trip to the doctor to get an exam, prescription for an antibiotic maybe some blood work to be sure as not serious as it would be for a sickle cell patient. After some medicine, lots of rest and liquid diets to stay hydrated if you lost your appetite soups will be your best friend but you will be better within a week.

When you have sickle cell getting a common cold or infection can be the start to more health issues if not caught in a timely manner. A fever of 101 degrees can be an automatic admittance and 48 hour stay to be sure that the sickle cell patient does not have any further issues the medical team will monitor you and treat pain. There are times when the doctor is not able to cure what is making your sick. When this happens we learn to control the symptoms or prevent them from getting worst.

Lee and his Sickle Cell also participates in research studies every once in a while to do his part in helping find a cure and understand what goes on when he has a pain episode. This helps the doctors find what triggers the problem and help Lee as well as others who have Sickle Cell. He realized that it goes with him everywhere and he always has to be aware so he wanted to help others see and understand what Sickle Cell Anemia is so he can bring awareness and do his part to help. If patients don't help by participating in some of the clinical trials the cure will never be discovered. When you volunteer for a study you are provided with expert medical treatment, current information, free lab and some compensation. With the computer capabilities in all our devices we can google sickle cell research, clinical trials, find local schools and the latest research activities in your community.

So I take care of my Sickle cell because it is a part of me. Sort of like you would attend to your pet. I have to keep it on a short leash sometimes because it misbehaves like when I get sick, except I don't feed my pet Sickle pet food I drink plenty of water to stay hydrated to help the blood flow easier and I eat healthy a basic diet but not so much fried foods. Really I can have the same diet as anyone what is bad for everyone is bad for me and can be a bit worst at times.

In the sickle cell community we have a way we remember to avoid issues called **F.A.R.M.S.**

F is for Fluids & Fever:

We must drink lots of water and pay attention to if we have a Fever. If over 101 we must see the doctor as soon as possible.

A is for Air:

Be sure to get enough oxygen especially in high altitudes, mountains, and planes.

R is for Rest:

Don't overdo it get plenty of sleep and take breaks when your body is tired.

M is for prevention Medicine:

Your daily medication like folic acid is needed to make new red blood cells or hydrea for pain prevention.

S is for Situations:

Avoid getting to cold or hot, avoid alcohol, illegal drugs, and smoking.

Following preventative measures is so important for children with sickle cell and drinking plenty of water can help a lot because kidneys are another organ that is damagedby the red blood cells that are sickled. The suggested amount of water you drink based onyour weight so if I weigh 30 pounds I should drink five to eight cups of water or if Iweighed 55 pounds I should drink about seven to ten eight ounce cups a day. Drinkingother fluid is okay like sports drinks, fruit juice, milk, and even soup is good. When it ishot popsicles are a real great treat but you will want to limit the soda, coffee, alcohol and highly caffeinated drinks like energy drinks. All of those drinks cause your kidneys to release more water in the your urine which can lead to dehydration faster so no more than two of the limited drinks per day is suggested. Check with your doctor to get your recommended water consumption per your specific body weight because too much of anything including water can cause your body harm.

FACT: The first sign of an infection is a fever and the parents need to be contacted immediately if the child's fever is over 101degrees. The most common infection to worry about is bacterial that can be the biggest risk for sickle cell children birth to five. Although at any age infections are serious and the spleen does not work as well in sickle cell patients so this makes it harder to fight them off. The spleen is the main defense system our body has against life threatening germs. So knowing the child's temperature is a vital clue to if there is an illness approaching and preventative measures should be taken.

2

School for a Kidd like me

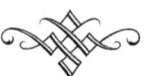

Lee headed towards his room and got dressed for school but he did not feel like his normal self this morning he was a little tired and wanted to stay at home. Determined to go to school because his class had done well on a test and won a pizza party today. So he grabbed his coat, slid his fingers in the gloves, put his hat on his head, and pulled his arms through the straps of his backpack heading out into the cold to catch the bus.

Lee learned to appreciate who he was and although he knew he had some limitations they weren't going to define him. Starting to pay attention he was learning what was good for him and what would cause his sickle cell to act up. One thing I found out is whatever you have that you have to take care of you need to understand it before you can help others. Like anything that requires responsibility there is a good and bad side. For some reason we all see the bad more I guess because it feels so horrible when it is happening to you. Well this is who Lee was and he cares for his sickle cell and others who have or are affected by it. Mostly because he has lived with it and it will be with him for his entire life until a cure is found that he can actually get.

FACT: Physical exhaustion can lead to a pain crisis if a child has difficulty carry textbooks allow them to use a rolling backpack or give them an extra set of books for home.

As his mother waved good-bye from the window she could not help but to be so protective. She always worried about him yet she liked to treat him just like the rest the children as much as she could. Raising her son gave her insight on what it is like to live with Sickle Cell. She looked at herself as not only his advocate but all of those who are affected by its advocate. She knows because she has seen the pain in her son's eyes and couldn't make it just go away by herself.

Being a mom of a child with an illness requires so much patience and strength on both the outside and inside. When he is unable to fight she puts on her boxing gloves and jumps in the ring for him. She has to also be able to know the difference between a basic cold, playing sick to get out of something, or a pain crisis. Yes, like every mom she is part detective and has eyes in the back of her head, she is part psychic, a chef, a nurse, a race car driver or chauffer, and at times she could join the circus with as many things as she juggles at once. That is her job and she accepts it with honor because it was not a challenge she could ever turn away from before accomplishing it and moving on to the next obstacle.

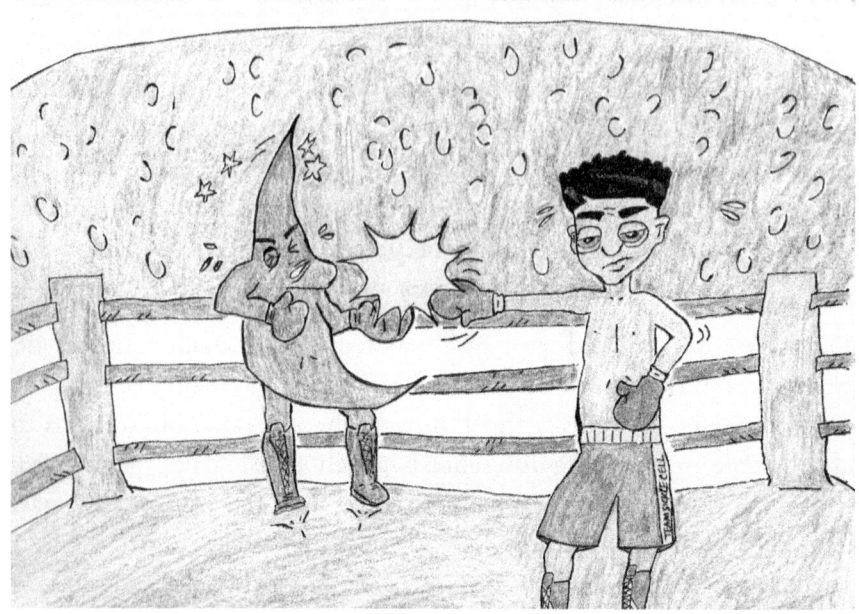

As Lee's mother she knows he is special and caring for him requires compassion while keeping him an equal. He still has chores, homework, and if he misbehaves he will still get put on punishment. No video games, no tv, no company, no fun so there are no special privileges or get out of jail free cards. It is important to treat him the same as his siblings so that there is peace among the family and he also has to understand this is real life. So when he gets in his I can't do this and poor me I'm sick mood because it is a test or chore that he has to attend to it is me who brings him to reality "Earth to Lee?.. Earth to Lee?" it is not happening like that buddy. It is important that he doesn't feel that rewards come with being sick. As a family we encourage and motivate to give him hope and strength when he is feeling down or sick and we all fight this together.

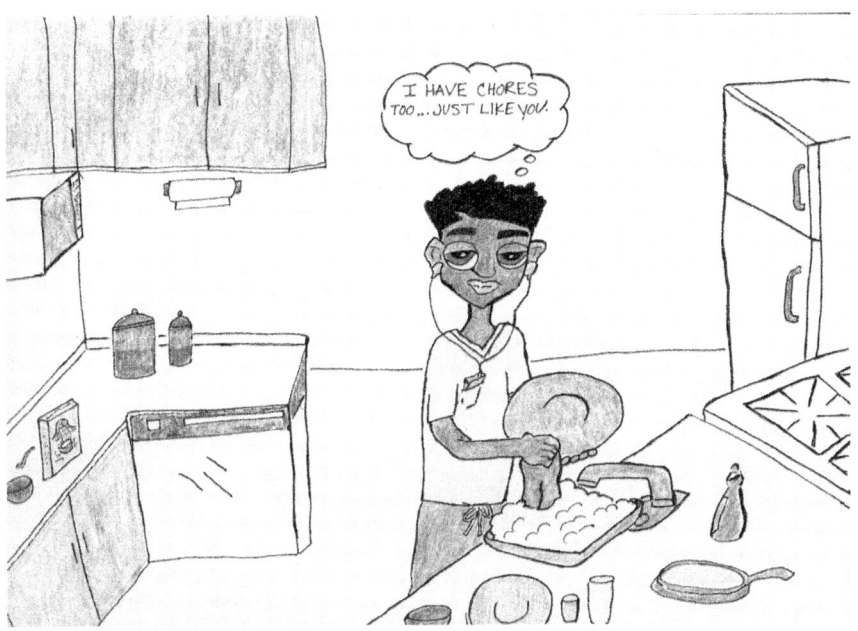

FACT: A child with sickle cell need to avoid extreme climate changes and temperatures that last long periods of time. In winter time they can not be in the cold for long periods of time. In the summer a person with sickle cell should take frequent breaks and drink lots of fluids to stay hydrated. Changes in temperature often should be avoided and controlled climates such as air conditioner and heater can cause complications that may lead to school absences or hospitalization.

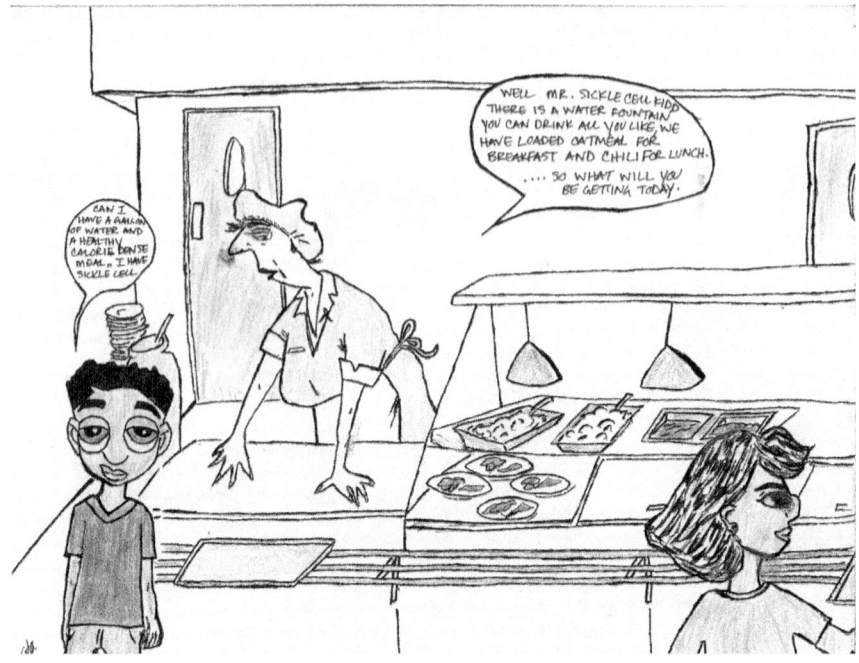

Getting off the school bus, Lee headed to the lunch room to get some breakfast or at least see if the cafeteria was serving something he likes. He decided to just grab some juice and a blueberry muffin. He headed to the table where he saw two of his buddies and took a seat next to his friend Jacob. They laughed and talked about the latest Dragon Ball Z episode when Thomas said "Lee, why are your eyes so yellow?" and Lee swallowed the juice that was in his mouth, lifted his brow and said, "Because I have secret super powers" his friend and him rose up from the table at the same time and tossed their trash.

That started a chain reaction because another boy asked in a sort of know it all voice from the end of the table "How come you are sick more than my cousin, he has a sickle cell trait? And he doesn't get sick all the time."

Lee sighed and shook his head, it is sad that there are so many misunderstanding about Sickle Cell. There are actually four common types of Sickle Cell and having a trait does not count as having the actual illness. Lee said, "Sickle Cell trait is when someone inherits just one normal hemoglobin "A" gene and one sickle gene. It is a very small and rare chance that they have complications because they did not inherit two Sickle Cell genes, they have a greater risk of serious complications if they going extreme in the sport, low oxygen and dehydration can start a backup of the blood in the spleen which could trigger a pain crisis even for them, but it is not that common."

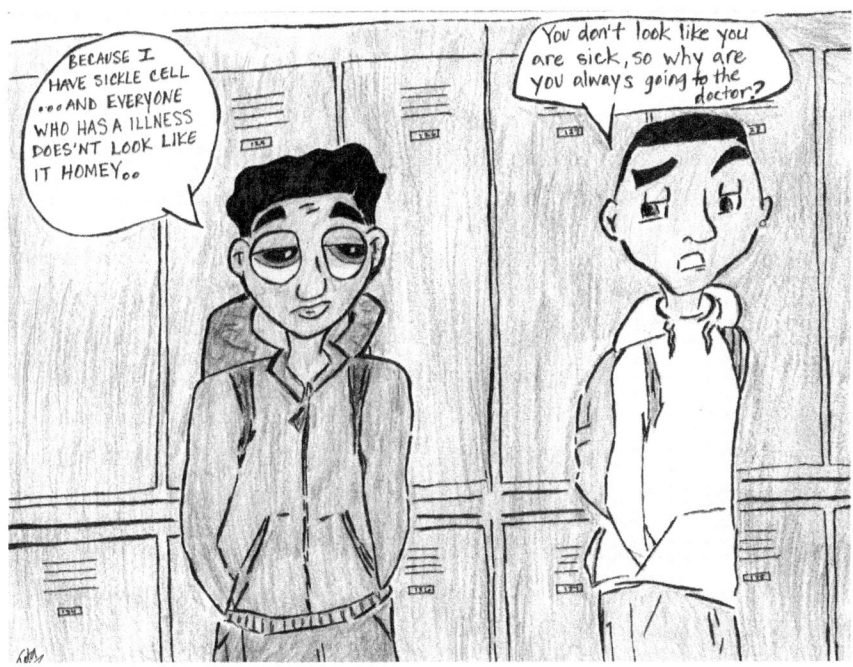

The boy sat on the end of the table with his eyebrows up in a scowl as if he had been given some new information and he still thought he knew more than he actually did. That is when Lee decided to give him a little bit more so he added, "Actually there are few types of Sickle Cell that affect people in different ways and they are sickle cell SC which is a milder case, then there is sickle cell SB which is more common in the United States due to huge number of Southeast Asia immigrants it causes no anemia or problems but combined with a hemoglobin problem thalassemia."

Next sickle cell SS which is what I have, which is caused from inheriting an S gene from both parents and that comes from both parents having a trait or the disease. This is a serious disease inherited anemia, causes organ damage, more infections, and pain crisis." Returning the matter of fact tone then Lee and his friends at the table got up and started to walk away but not before he turned around to add, "I hope you learned something new today". They all huddled in a group as they ran out the cafeteria.

Yelling from behind the counter "No running in the cafeteria!" the lunch lady said. So Lee and his friend Jacob slowed down into a sort of power walk. Lee could see his teacher at the door of his classroom.

"How are you doing today Lee?" asked Ms. Bosswell. "I'm fine, thanks for asking" Lee replied. Lee walked over to his cubby and removed his coat, scarf, and hat. He rolled his backpack to his chair removed his gloves and stuck them in the pocket of his backpack and pulled out a bottle of water then sat it on his desk. He hung his backpack on the back of the chair as he took his seat. His teacher Ms. Boswell closed the class door and she turned around to greet her class with a smile.

Mrs. Bosswell knew Lee had Sickle Cell and she recalled a friend when she was in who had the disease when she was in grade school and remembered that she was so fragile and sickly. She had her good days and bad days but Mrs. Boswell thought it was basically a low iron problem for a long time until she read the packet that Lee's mom brought in when he started her class. His mom also gave a packet to the front office and his gym teacher so that they were all aware of the precautions to take and what to do if a problem occurs. It is very important for parents to inform the school of any health issues with the students because the school is their home away from home.

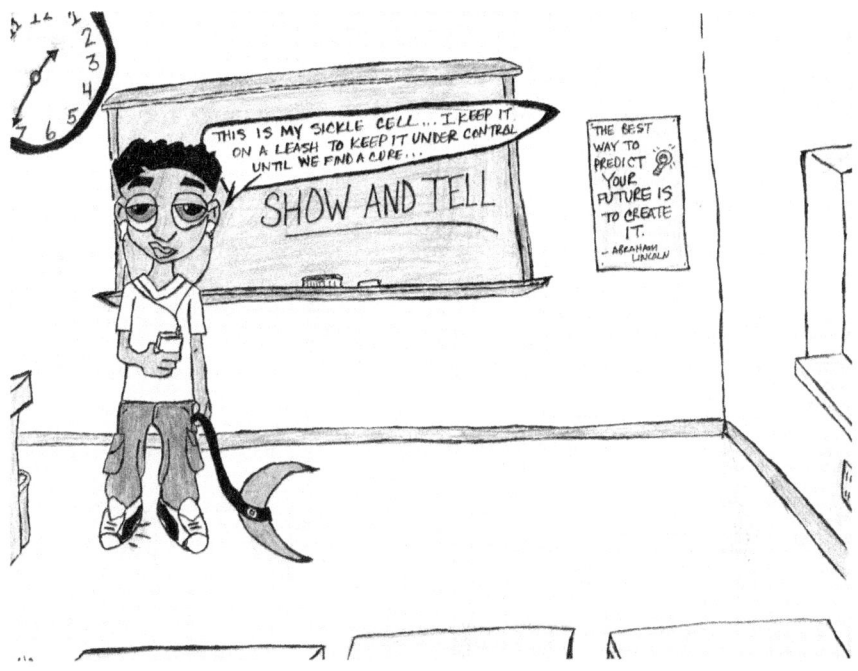

FACT: The child has to be given plenty of fluids and must have them available to them at all times in class. They should be allowed to carry a water bottle at all times and to drink water during class, during physical education (P.E) or any other time. This is because children fluids assist red blood cells in moving more easily through the blood vessels, which will decrease the amount of pain crises the children may experience. This also means that they should have free access to the bathroom because children with sickle cell need to go to the bathroom more often due to their high fluid intake and, their kidney do not function as well as the healthy children.

"Good morning, boys and girls" in a slight melody the class replied, "Good Morning Ms. Boswell". The teacher walked over to her desk and began to take the attendance and then she looked up from her notebook and asked for everyone to pass their homework forward. The class filled with the sound of zippers opening, papers ruffling and the room filled with the hum of chatter about the hope that everyone completed did their homework because the deal was if everyone not only completed their homework but received a passing grade the class could have a pizza party and a movie.

As Ms. Boswell walked by each row she picked up four papers with the grand total of twenty, which meant that everyone turned in their homework. She smiled and announced "Alright class, it seems like everyone has submitted their homework, and that's great. So take out your reading books, turn to chapter eleven, and start reading while I grade your papers." The class began to surge with sighs and that's when Ms. Boswell said "Excuse me but the room should be silent during reading."

Looking up from his book Lee glanced at the clock for the fourth time. He counts the minutes and realizes that it has been fifty-four minutes and he was on the nineteenth page in the chapter. As he looked around the class he noticed that he wasn't the only one getting antsy. Then the clock read 9:30 am and right at that moment Ms. Boswell rolled her chair back away from her desk and stood up. She walked over to the board and began writing then turned around and stepped away from the board revealing the words "All passed". The students burst into cheer.

"Alright, settle down class. Now since today is our minimum day we will have to get this party started at eleven o'clock." Holding a stack of papers in her hand Ms. Bosswell she began passing out a work packet for the weekend for chapter eleven. She told everyone to get in their work groups and finish reading the chapter and then start on the work packet, which will be due on Monday.

So everyone went to their assigned groups, time went by really fast because before Lee could get to the second worksheet there was Ms. Boswell walking in with five pizzas and fried chicken buffalo wings. She pulled out a case of water and soda along with plates and cups.

Once everyone was seated back with their pizza, wings and drink Ms. Boswell pushed the television to the front of the classroom and cut on the movie.

FACT: Eating a balanced diet, a healthy diet. Drinking plenty of fluids will prevent dehydration but eating greasy foods and not drinking enough fluids can trigger a pain crisis.

By the time the movie was over they only had fifteen minutes left in class so Lee had to get his belongings and get ready to board the bus. Lee started to feel tired so he wasn't moving as fast as he wanted to but he hurried off to board his bus and get a good seat. His stop was not to far from the school and Lee could not wait to get off the bus and get home. As he was getting off his stop he could see his mom waiting at the bus stop and he walked up to her and gave her a hug.

"Hey baby, how was your day?" said Lee's mom. "It was good, we had a pizza party and watched a movie because everyone did their homework with a passing grade." said Lee. "Well that sounds like you had a good day" said his mom as they walked to their house. Lee walked in his room and threw his backpack on the floor in the corner near his bookshelf. His stomach was feeling a little funny so he went to the restroom and then he decided to lay down for a little bit. About two hours passed Lee had been asleep and he woke from a sharp pain so he got up, went straight to the restroom again but this time he was in pain all of a sudden which is common with sickle cell anemia.

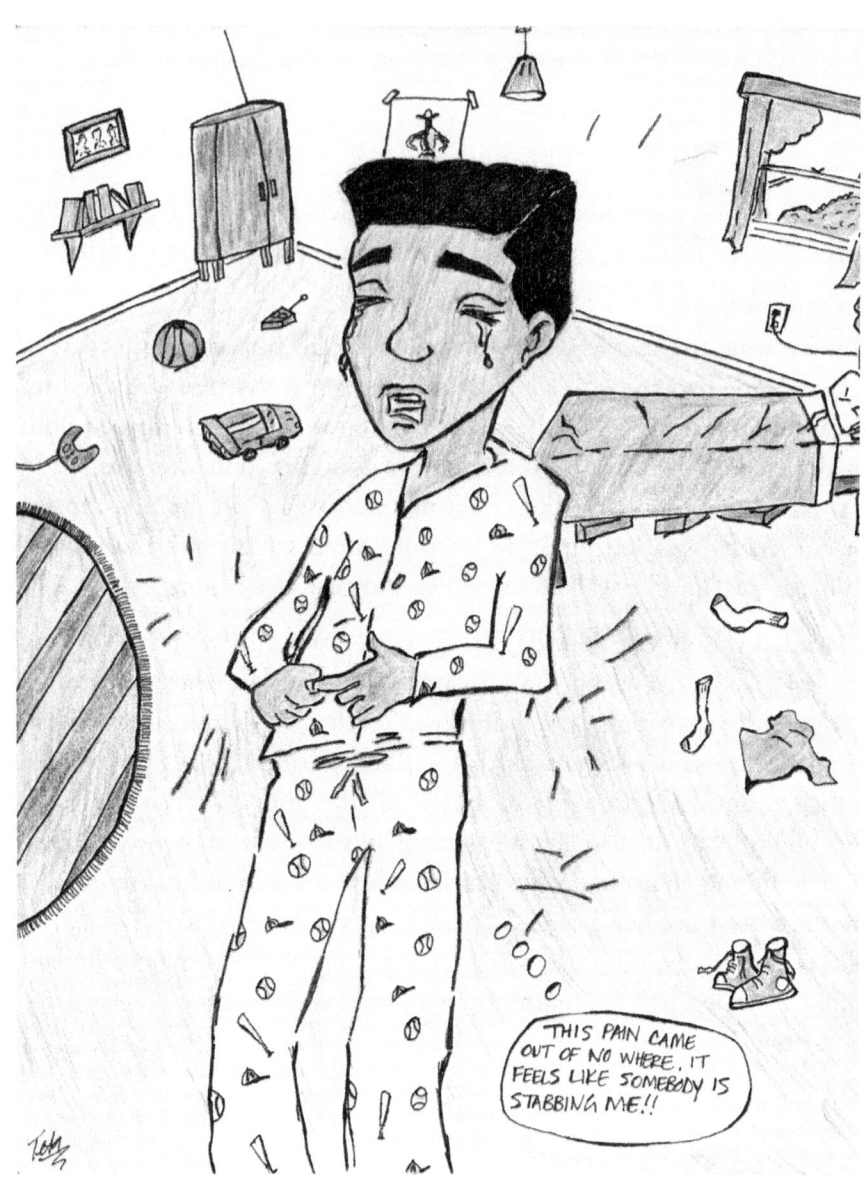

FACT: The three most common type of Sickle Cell disease are hemoglobin SS disease (also known as sickle cell anemia), hemoglobin SC disease and sickle cell beta thalassemia.

3

Hold my hand through this

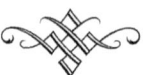

Pain episodes can come on very quickly. Some patients go a long time without any episodes but others can have a few episodes a month. There are triggers that bring on a crisis like dehydration, stress, fever, low oxygen, chilly or very hot temperatures to name a few. Often pain crisis targets the arms, back, legs, stomach, chest, and even the head.

Nothing is more significant than the family and patient being able to distinguish the clues a sickle cell crisis has once complications surface out of nowhere. This is when all of the preparations need to be used all noticing the sickle cell features that basically show during a typical pain episode that can be maintained at home. If the pain lasts longer than usual, or if the pain increases and the patient goes from able to talk to unable to walk in a short span of time it is time to seek urgent medical attention. We use a pain scale, one being the lowest level of pain and ten being the highest this is a communication tool to monitor how the patient feels and if it is progressing or not.

Lee didn't want to cry but he was in pain and he didn't want to worry his mom. Before he could call out for help his brother knocked on the door and asked was he okay. Hearing how Lee was sounded through the door his older brother ran to get his mom. She rushed to the bathroom door, picked the lock then rushed to Lee's side and began other pain methods like sitting him in a warm bath, meditation or listening to music are a few things that helps him calm down as she called his hematologist. Lee has a poem that he says as the pain hits him he recites this through the pain.

Make this pain go away, I have faith and so I pray

Very soon I will be okay, to sing and play

Another day

It was after hours so the answering service paged the doctor on call and while they waited for the doctor his mom took his temperature, which read 101 degrees and that is an automatic trip to the emergency room, so Lee's mom started to get him ready to go to the hospital. She gave him some Ibuprofen his dad decided to stay at home with his brother and sister then they headed to the hospital.

On the drive to the hospital as Lee laid on the backseat of his mom's car he started to go to his place where he stops thinking about his pain but he knew his mom was right there that also helps him cope with the pain. Pulling up to the emergency room they were met by the valet.

FACT: With a fever of 101 degrees is bad for anyone but is really bad a person with sickle requires immediate attention from a doctor to see if there is an infection and give them medication that can get to the system quicker through an IV (intravenously).

Providing basic Sickle Cell education for all the members of the immediate family, and caregivers is very important. Understanding when to go to the hospital and what is causing the pain is very necessary. This is the key that unlocks doors of silence or shame that the child or family feels when the child is in pain, sick often, admitted to the hospital, misses school, and can't participate in some activities. It is important to make them feel as normal as possible and comfortable enough to not be ashamed or scared to tell you or someone that they are in pain. This gives them reassurance and confidence in themselves and those who they will count on to take care of them. The hugs and love go a very long way when you are dealing with an illness it all matters as well as helps to ease the pain and silence the fear inside.

Closing his yellow eyes briefly through the pain he is met by his nurse she said her name was Cindy. She asks Lee "on a scale from 1 to 10, how bad is the pain?" Lee thought briefly and said "6". Nurse Cindy walked over to the cart picked up the angio catheter, Lee thinks it looks like a butterfly it is for an IV to start giving Lee some fluids through his veins this is to help him with dehydration.

Lee made it in time to beat the pain and regain his strength. His hematology team is at his side and ready to get him back to 100 percent. This is done through hooking Lee up to machines an IV, oxygen, taking needed medicine, and getting some rest. Lee was twisting his special identification bracelet he received when he arrived to the hospital for security reasons this must be worn at all times. Lee began visualizing his strength this is a form of meditation because it helps him take his mind off the pain although the pain is fading away he can still feel it. He was going to stay for 1 to 2 days because he had a high fever which could mean an infection and he wasn't too happy about that but he has his family who keeps him strong, and focused on healing.

FACT: Chronic pain is the other type the doctor will name and this lasts for a weeks to months and can be really hard to take and this could really limit the regular daily activities.

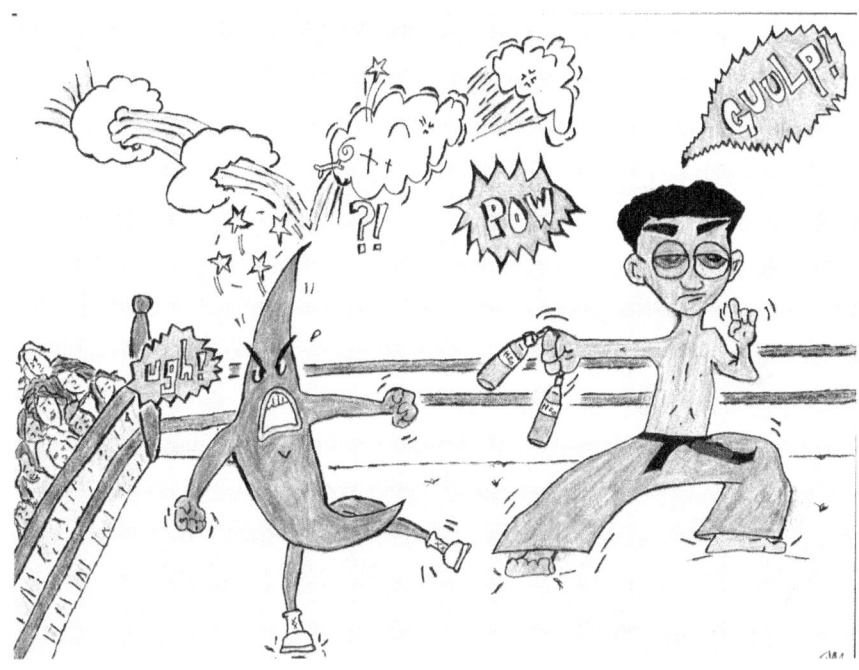

The pain has gone down some and even though there is a sharp feeling Lee still finds strength to laugh at a joke on the show he was watching while resting in bed. Staying positive keeps Lee's attitude out of the darkness it also gives him a way to cope with the pain. These are other ways Lee fights his sickle cell and the pain it brings. If he isn't hydrated enough it creates a great environment for a crisis to occur this will make one of his triggers go off because the cells are like liquid fiber, they get stiff, and caught in the blood vessels. Doing all of that it makes the blood flow unable to get to all of the organs with the oxygen needed to work properly and it can cause pain. It is like when a pet is acting up chewing the wires to your video game, or your shoes. Lee's Sickle Cell is disciplined by a good diet, staying hydrated, his medication, and knowing his limits.

Well say hello to sickle cell he creates crisis in Lee's body because they change their shape into a "C" and only last about 10 to 20 days. That is not very long compared to the normal red blood cells that are round and last about 120 days in the bloodstream they both carry oxygen and remove carbon dioxide (waste product) from your body.

FACT: The red blood cells are made in the spongy marrow inside large bones of the body. Bone marrow is always producing new red blood cells so they can replace the old ones but the bone marrow can't make the new ones fast enough to replace the sickle cells that don't last as long. Folic acid is a vitamin that helps the body produce new red blood cells.

Lee has yellow eyes and that is part of his identity that is not a secret anymore. He has a sidekick that he was born with and that is Sickle Cell. Together they are one, fighting an ongoing battle in this world of health. Like any superhero Lee has a mask but that mask is a special one that gives him oxygen. He does not wear it all of the time but he uses it when he needs to. It is important for those who Lee has contact with know how he is special and what he needs to prevent a crisis as well as how to handle one when it occurs. The hematology team is a special team that helps Lee return to full power.

Nurse Cindy came into his room to give an update to Lee's mom letting her know that Lee was doing much better and will probably be able to go home this afternoon. Once admitted the nurses asked him a series of questions and ran a few tests. Nurse Cindy noticed Lee said after the pizza party he did not feel well. Lee said he ate some pizza and a few pieces of fried chicken. That made her think he should possibly be tested for gallstones being a hematology nurse she has seen the similar symptoms on other sickle cell patients. Carrying that important piece of information to the team was a key factor in finding the source to Lee's pain crisis.

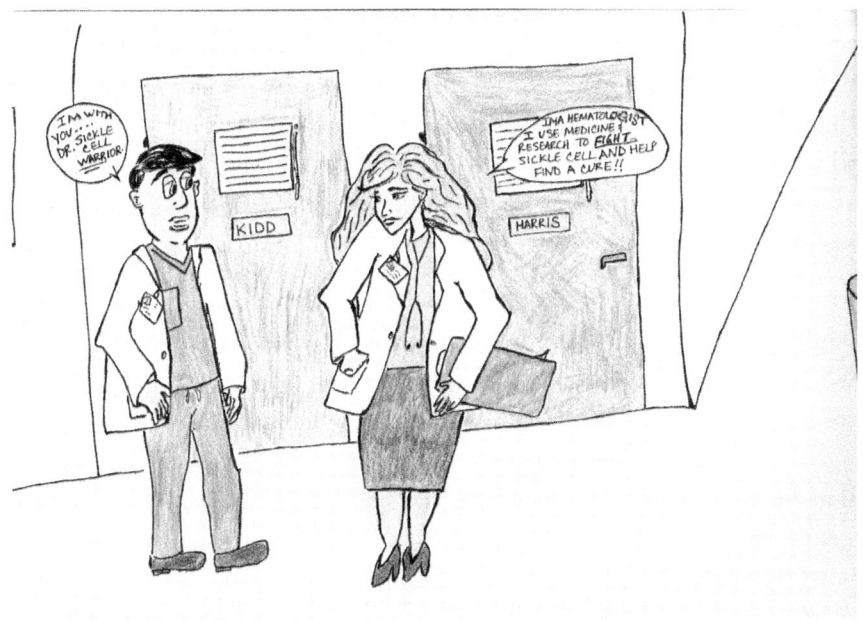

This was good news because Lee would normally have to stay at least two days longer if he was any sicker and didn't recover as fast. His family worked as a team and saw the signs that Lee was going into a pain episode. They made him feel better until he could get to the hospital and see his doctor to get his pain treated. Dr. Green walked in with the final diagnosis that Lee did in fact have gallstones which come from the red blood cells breaking apart and they make more bile stones (bile helps your body digest fatty foods) with sickle cell has increased red cell hemolysis) which causes nausea, pain in the stomach, and greasy foods are a major trigger. With that being discovered his team scheduled for Lee to have a surgery to have his gallbladder removed.

"Surgery!" yelled Lee his heart began to beat faster anxiety started to kick in until he heard Dr. Green voice through his clouded imagination. "Now, Lee this is a very common surgery that sickle cell patients have and you will get to meet with the surgeon and ask him all the questions you want." said Dr. Green in a reassuring voice. So the nurse came in and gave them an appointment to come and have a consultation about the surgery and then schedule the procedure. Lee felt confident that he would be able to go through with the surgery and he knew that his family and his medical team were there to help him be healthy so with that information he put his smile back on his face looked over at his mom and said "I am not scared I am glad I know what was making me sick now and we can fix it".

Most heroes have a special team that helps keep their identity a secret while they save the world. Lee is not that kind of hero he decided he would be the hero who would not hide behind the mask he wanted to tell people about his battles and give them courage to stand up and fight whatever challenges ahead of them. Having sickle cell Lee knows that his team helps him reach his full capacity it just so happens that Lee's team is made up of his doctors, nurses, therapists, specialist, and with them combined they are his "Hematology Team".

Smiling at her son Lee's mom looked over at him thinking he was so strong and he always kept such a positive attitude. If he only knew that made her stronger and kept her fighting for him every day. Meanwhile on the inside Sickle Cell was approached by folic acid that brought on some new red blood cells to bring that good oxygen to all of Lee's organs and limbs. Oxygen, fluids, and medicine to stop the pain all makes Sickle behave. There is always some pain in this battle to get through the bloodstream when sickle cells block the flow through the small blood vessels. Drinking plenty of fluids can lower risks for a painful crisis and when in the hospital having an IV gets the fluids in Lee's system much faster. The doctor finally came in saying that Lee had some acute pain which is more common and happens all of a sudden it also can range from mild to severe it lasts for hours or up to a few days. The doctor said that Lee needs to continue his medication and he can go home because he is back at full power and ready to fight again.

While Lee's mom gathered all of his belongings, his nurse prepared the discharge papers and he started to get dressed and ready to go home.

Monday he thought that he would return to school and tell his closest friends about his latest battle. Lee recalled when he stayed with his dad while his mom was getting settled in a new state during his parents' divorce and he went on a field trip to the beach. His dad Freddie was getting used to handling his care and all the things that could trigger a crisis but he didn't think too much about him going on an overnight to field trip to Pier 39 with his entire class. Who could resist living the life of a sailor for a day, getting their feet wet and sand between their toes? Lee joined his friends after visiting the Pier getting up early like a sailor feeling the cool ocean air while they all ran to the beach although it was chilly but he figured he would only get his feet wet. The water was freezing but he ran along the shore for a while with his classmates before long it was time to go gather his things, get back on the bus and head home.

On the ride home his feet started to hurt and when he got home he was in a full blown crisis, his feet had swollen some, and they hurt badly. On the bus he tried to pretend he was alright but his friends saw he was in pain and told his teacher who told his father. So his dad rushed him to the emergency room and they told him he was having a pain crisis called the hand/foot syndrome. His father was able to handle his pain episode by taking him to get immediate medical care. He contacted Lee's mom to let her know of the latest pain crisis and that he was alright. He was so used to the questions from his classmates, friends and even family so he tried his best not to let the questions of those who don't understand make him feel bad. Instead Lee let people know how it is from his experience and give them a chance to see this illness through his yellow eyes.

Fact: There are things that can be done to prevent a crisis from occurring such as drinking lots of water. It dilutes the blood and helps keep the amount of sickled cells pretty low. Having a transfusion which gives new blood cells or infusion which takes out bad blood and replaces it with more good blood does that as well. Avoiding places or situations that expose him to low oxygen levels like sports competitions, or boot camp. Staying out of high altitudes like flying long periods of time, mountain climbing, or living in cities with high altitudes or in mountains will help avoid a crisis.

4

Taking care of yourself

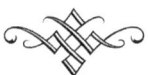

To stay healthy with sickle cell there are frequent doctor appointments to attend. Lots of tests are done during those visits to monitor not only the sickle cell but also the other complications that come from having the pain episodes. Remember earlier in the book I mentioned that Lee has pain episodes that cause damage to his organs and tissue. Routine appointments are to monitor his illness while those appointments are usually a few hours of all the tests that have to be ran are done during that time.

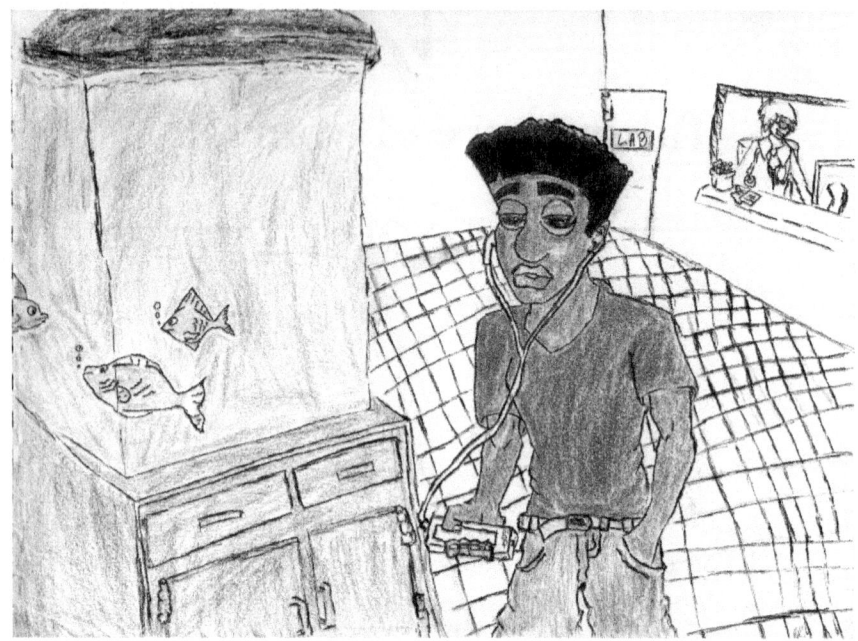

Going to get lab work done is not so bad, a complete blood count (CBC) shows your medical team how your blood cells are doing by measuring an important counted section of the red blood cells complete blood volume. The CBC is a few blood test all at once for white blood cells, platelets, and red blood cells. Lee is asked to pee in a cup for a urinalysis to make sure his kidney is working correctly and urine protein test to make sure that the is not too much protein being released by his kidney in the urine. The kidney shows the first sign of damage by releasing protein in your urine. There are about eight more tests like eye exams, hearing tests, x-rays, exercise tests to measure how the lungs and hearts are working, six minute walk exam on a long hallway to see how fast you can walk back and forth 100 feet.

All of the tests play a vital role in the care for Lee and anyone with sickle cell anemia to assist in finding any brain damage early bone damage and other particular infections. Now there are some very important tests that give a special view of what is going on inside on the body. A computerized tomography scan (CT Scan) lets the doctor see a cross-section view of the organs in your body which can find blockages, blood, growths, swelling, stroke, and tumors. A picture taken of the blood vessels and organs inside the body is called a magnetic resonance imaging (MRI).

One of the tests is called a transcranial doppler (TCD) it sounds funny and maybe a little scary but it does not hurt at all. It is an ultrasound test for the brain that measures how fast and disorderly the blood is flowing through the blood vessels to get to it. For children with sickle cell this is the best way the hematology team can foretell a possibility of the child's first stroke. Due to sickle cell damage many blood vessels can partially or fully close over which creates a blockage. It is sort of like when your pipes in your house are blocked by debris which lead to erosion causes you to loose water pressure.

Lee had an appointment today and he was having a TCD scan done so he knew that he would be getting to see a picture inside of his own head which was exciting. He knew that this test was to see if he would be likely to have a stroke or not because he has this test done since he was three years old and when Lee tested moderate or conditional he was scheduled to have another TCD scan within two months. With results of moderate or conditional to high risk means the child is likely to have a stroke. Staying on top of all of the doctor appointments is a job because if an important test is scheduled during that appointment it will cause a delay on diagnosing the problem and it may be too late to prevent some of the worst outcomes.

Both parents are in Lee's life but he stays with his mom mostly because his parents are divorced now but they still get along especially when it comes to family situations. There are times when Lee's older brother Angel would babysit while their mom worked and so they all had a routine on those days. On one particular day their mom had to work late so the kids knew how to make a frozen dinner or heat up left overs so that is what they did. They called to check in when they got home from school and all went on to their normal after school routines. Lee had come home after his older brother who was already in the kitchen with his head half in the refrigerator in search for an after school meal.

Lee had a bad headache so he wanted to just go and lay down feeling kind of weak and dizzy he grabbed a seat at the table. "Hey Big head" said Angel to Lee as he poked his head from out of the freezer as he searched for food. In a dragging tone Lee replied "Heeeyy?" and as he heard himself he realized that he sounded funny, I guess his brother noticed he said it funny too because he laughed out loud and said "Why did you say it like that?" as he walked out of the kitchen he gave Lee a playful punch to his right arm and it tingled like it fell asleep or something.

Using the rail as he walked upstairs to his room Lee had this weak feeling but he thought he was tired and so he went in his room took off his school clothes and put on his pajamas. Looking at the tree outside his window the leaves were blowing Lee couldn't help but think it was a nice day outside. The sun lit his room and it would be hard to fall asleep any other time but it did not seem to bother him at all because before he could turn his blinds his eyes were shut. Opening his eyes Lee realized he was sleep for a while the room was lit only by the light from the tv. It was dark and he felt like he slept wrong because his whole right side was numb he looked up at the window and saw it was a half-moon outside. The shadow from the tree crawled across his walls as if reaching for him that made a chill run down his back so he tried to sit straight up and he felt like he was stuck and then he started to slowly move but it felt tingly all over his right side.

Lee stood up, walked to his door and opened it and he could hear music coming from his sister Minnie's room so he knew she was home. Rushing up the stairs Minnie saw Lee walking towards the bathroom and she was going to have to beat him to it. "Move Lee!! I gotta go really bad and Angel is downstairs stinking up the other one!" she yelled. She flew in the bathroom and slammed the door behind her leaving Lee standing at the top of the stairs with some real smart big brother comment he had hanging on the tip of his tongue ready to throw at her like darts but he could not get the words to come out. Annoyed Lee walked downstairs into the den sat on the couch to watch some cartoons when Angel came out the bathroom asking what he was watching Lee looked at over to him and he said "Blue" hearing what just came out his mouth Lee laughed and so did Angel although there was something off they were always being silly so there was no second thoughts.

Minnie came in playing around as usual and tossed a pillow at Lee while he was watching cartoons like a zombie. Mom had already made dinner and gone to bed she worked a twelve hour shift and when she got in she made some spaghetti and garlic rolls then off to bed she went. Minnie told Lee his plate was in the microwave and he said "I don't want breakfast" and both Angel and Minnie looked at Lee and busted out laughing. Minnie said "It's s-p-a-g-h-e-t-t-i not BREAKFAST you play too much!" and Lee laugh turned into a giggle and he shook his head and said "I know ..Brreaakf-a-s-s-s-s-t". Then they all giggled but Lee heard himself and he stopped laughing. Angel jumped up off the couch and looked at Lee asking him if he was okay? Lee slowly stopped smiling with a look of confusion he felt tears filling his eyes he nodded although a tear slipped out his eye falling down his cheek.

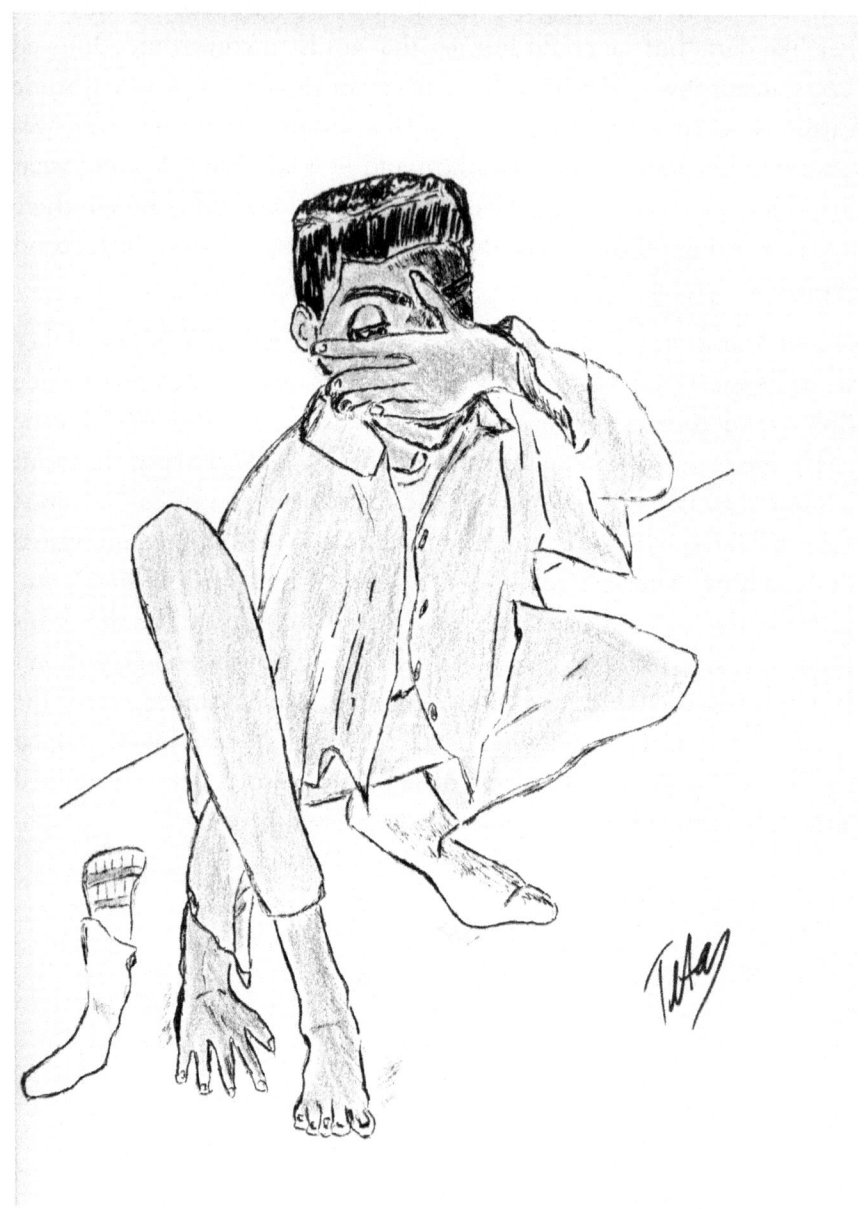

"GO GET MOM!" Angel yelled at Minnie who turned to run up the stairs to tell mom that something is wrong with Lee. Jumping out of her sleep their mom heard someone burst in her room and Minnie flicked the switch and the room exploded with light. Sitting straight up her heart racing being woke out of a dead sleep after working a double shift she saw her daughter looking as if she was terrified. Talking a mile a minute she was shouting, "Something is wrong with Lee! He is talking funny and we were laughing then he started crying because he couldn't say spaghetti right! He kept saying breakfast! There is something wrong mom?.." Minnie blurted out all in the same sentence with tears in her eyes so the mom knew that something was wrong. Rushing down to her son the mom could only begin going down her symptoms of sickle cell and the reasons mental checklist. The diagnosis that kept lingering in the back of her head was her son was having or had a stroke and she had to get him to the emergency room as soon as possible.

Grabbing the flashcard that was on the desk in the family room she sat next to Lee and told Angel to get his brother things together so we can go to the doctor just to be safe. She did not want to alarm her other children with her feared diagnosis of a stroke but she needed to get all of them to the car or call 9-1-1 being that he was sitting up and trying to communicate, and he could walk she made the decision to get them in the car and drive to the nearest emergency room. Flipping through the flashcards Lee's mom stopped and held up the "A card for Apple" and he said that, she held up "B card for Ball" he said that also so she felt better, so she held up "C for Cat" and Lee felt more confident when he said "DOG!" he laughed nervously and his mom said to stop laughing it's not funny and then Lee put his head down and started to cry.

They had been on countless trips down the highway to get to the emergency room at the Children's Hospital where they had a special blood disorder clinic with a sickle cell unit. This trip was different it seemed like they were floating on the highway as she made sure she stayed within the speed limit her car skated through traffic all the way to the hospital exit. Changing lanes she would catch a glance at her children holding their brother in the back seat fighting back the tears she gripped her steering wheel and hit her blinker. Calling ahead when she was loading the children in the car the hospital was aware they would be arriving with a possible stroke from a sickle cell patient who is already STAT (high priority) in the Emergency Room.

After checking Lee in with the triage nurse, he was taken to get an MRI done and it was determined that Lee in fact had a stroke which affected his right sided and his speech. This is known as dysphasia and aphasia is a common condition which is knowing what people are reading, saying, or writing but affects how you find the right words to say in reply. To treat a stroke a sickle cell patient is given a blood transfusion and if the TCD scan showed Lee was highly likely to have a stroke he could have started the transfusions preventatively. This is known as transfusion therapy which treats priapism and splenic sequestration as well as acute chest syndrome.

FACT: Arteries leading to the brain need oxygen and if a portion of the flow of blood that is rich in oxygen is blocked from the brain a stroke will occur. A stroke is one of the top five causes of death and the main cause of disability in the United States.

This was a serious life threatening situation which caused a setback for Lee because he had to learn basic skills of living again like talking, writing, responding to questions correctly. He was on intensive care unit for four days and then he was able to be transferred to the rehabilitation unit. Lee's father stays in another state but with technology they were able to face time, skype so it was like he was there with us for a visit when he called to check on Lee which brightened his day tremendously. Social media was the branch of communication for all of the family and friends which helped reading all of the uplifting prayers and reassurance. For thirty days we stayed at the hospital leaving for the little hours I could get a babysitter for the younger children luckily it was summer time so they did not miss any school. As for my job well I exhausted all of the FMLA, personal time off, until I eventually was laid off but that did not matter to me for that moment my only concern was my son and my family.

Being an artistic family Lee's mom brought in a MP3 player which had all his favorite hip hop songs downloaded, art supplies, and papers so they could draw which is something they would do anyway as a family. With his playlist on repeat Lee would be listening to his music unable to say the words but his body would rock to the beat and soon that led to him humming then words saying a few bars of the song. Before he could get discharged Lee was dancing around the rehab rapping to his music overcoming all obstacles he worked on his speech his way along with the speech therapist who actually invited his family to his sessions at times. The therapist had a modern approach and would use each patient's interests in a part of their therapy. The arts can be a huge tool for rehabilitation on any level it allows a person to express themselves when words can't be articulated.

In rehab Lee had to participate in occupational therapy to learn the daily life skills like motor skills for writing, self-care, he also had a physical therapist to help him regain his strength on his right side and a speech therapist to help with his speech due to aphasia. He would see them every day while he was in the hospital for a scheduled time which was part of his occupational therapy stay on schedule. It was bitter sweet on his last day because he made some great friends who was fighting their own health battles, he also had some great therapists who all knew him.

With his upbeat attitude always smiling even when he isn't feeling his best he won the hearts of the entire rehab staff. So they through Lee a graduating rehab party filled with all of the friends he made on his journey through rehab as well as all the therapists who took the time to explain what he was going through. His hematology team even made their way to the party for a few hugs so they all circled the room for Lee to go around saying how he had impacted the rehabilitation unit with his confidence and magnetic personality they all shared there good byes.

Now Lee has to have exchange transfusions that take the sickled blood cells from him while transfusing the donated red blood cells to prevent the sickled red blood cells from getting high. This is what they did when Lee had his stroke as well to decrease the amount of sickled hemoglobin in his system. There is no need to worry the transfusions are safe but there are significant issues that can happen relating to receiving transfusions such as alloimmunization which is common it occurs to a quarter of sickle cell patients who are transfused. This causes the donor blood to be attacked by the patient's immune system which delays the autoantibodies and the response to the transfusion so it makes it hard to find a donor with blood that is equal.

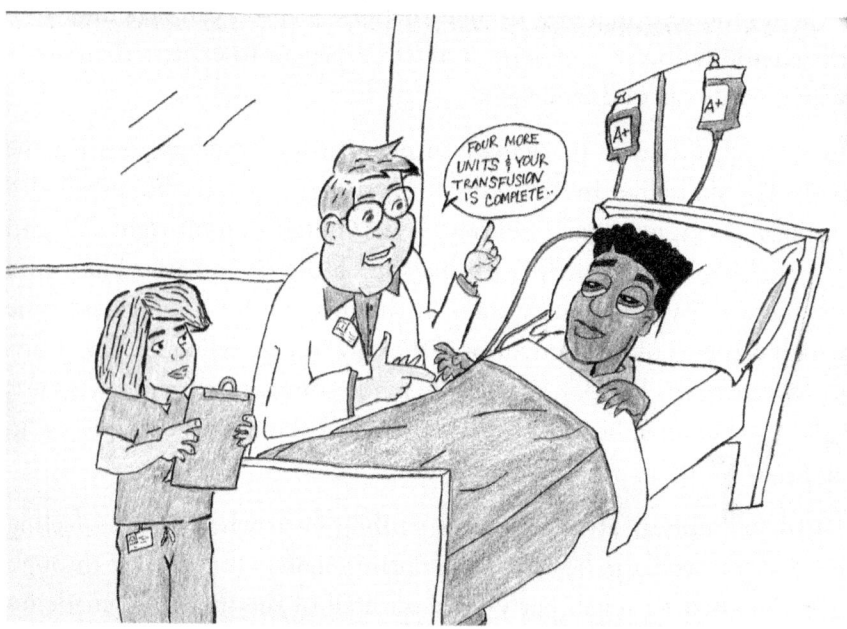

By doing a transfusion too quick a sickle cell patient can get a fluid overload because the body did not have time to adapt to the additional fluid and red blood cells. This can lead to a pain crisis or even a stroke because the blood gets to flow slow and gets thick. Be sure if either of these things happen to document it so it can help prevent any future reactions.

5

How to survive sickle cell

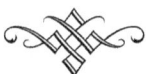

Getting back on his routine was going to be a challenge Lee thought he had just overcame some of his biggest fears having sickle cell he always knew that he had limits on everything that he could do. He would listen when the doctors would say what could happen if he has another stroke or stop getting his transfusions his entire life he was scared inside when he heard a new situation that his sickle cell can cause to happen to him. One thing Lee knew even as a young child is that he had his family and he was strongest with them. Having his stroke as a teenager was hard because he was not able to go to school, play sports, attend dances and most of the time he would brush it off but when he heard his friends talk about their experiences he could not help to wonder what it would be like to just be a regular kid in high school preparing for driving and graduation.

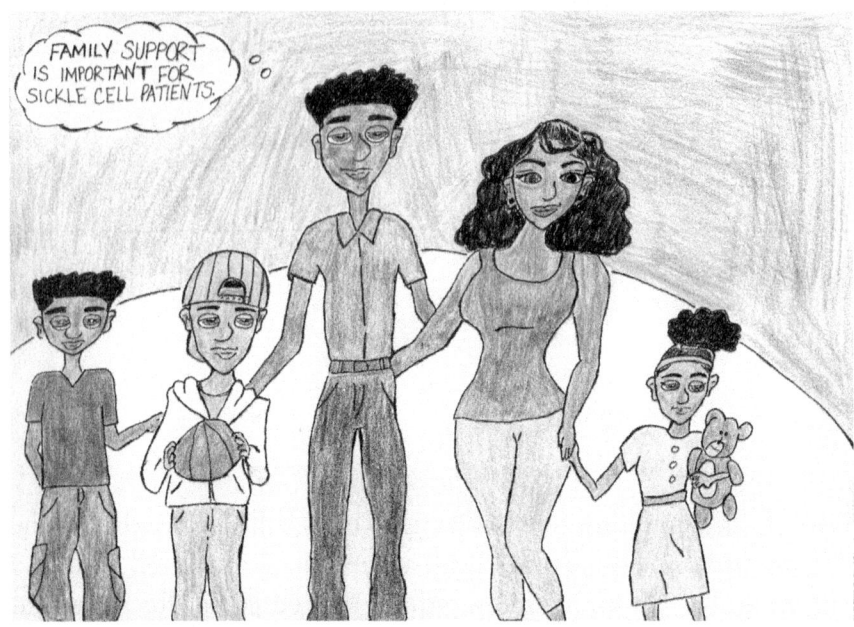

After a few months Lee had to make a decision about getting a port surgically put in his body. He had to get so many samples of blood drawn and had been stuck in so many places that thinking in the future he would have veins that would be unusable and hard. A port is a plastic catheter that is put in the large vein in the chest or arm under the skin with a chamber the size of a quarter that seals itself this allows the medical team to have the ability to have a reliable access point to give IV fluids, medications, blood and get samples of blood. It's alarming at first to think of a device being put inside of you knowing how it help save your veins and if a sickle cell patient has ever been hospitalized they know how many times you can be poked or your vein can give out. So having a port that requires only one needle prick is worth it.

Eventually you will have to get another port because the cans get infected or clotted so be sure that they are properly flushed out and cleaned each time it is used or handled. Lee's mom watched over the nurses as they cared for her son but she also taught him to ask questions and verify that something was or was not done. All sterile methods should be used anytime anyone is dealing with the port one key thing you can ask them as they are flushing your port if the solution is a weak form of heparin to stop the blood from clotting within the tube. Make sure when you are dealing with any other healthcare worker that they have handled a port before and they know what type of needles to use as well as the proper sterile techniques to prevent any other complications.

After all he had to overcome he wondered if a regular kid could handle all of the doctor appointments, getting poked; drained of blood, tested for every possible thing that could go wrong for someone who has sickle cell anemia. Lee knew ultimately it was his illness and he looked back at all the years his mother balanced her life, a job, and his care and wondered if she really was a superhero. He always saw her as growing up coming to save the day even if it hurt her she would do what she had to do for us he knew that for a fact. Lee had grown into a young man now having the stroke caused him to slip into isolation when he got home out of fear of talking in public and someone noticing his slur of words at times. He was still going to speech therapy talking was not so hard to overcome but seeing your friends who you were in school with driving and moving on to college can have anyone feeling a little depressed. Lee talked to his family friends there are times that you don't want to talk to them and his mom understood that so she found a few support groups through the sickle cell teen clinic program even online chat groups are great.

Being resourceful is what got our family through a lot of the hard times so contacting the local human resource center or disability benefit programs to find out if your particular medical condition sickle cell and/or stroke qualifies you for any of those programs. The internet is a great tool that we have now and there are countless articles on sickle cell if you type in the specific question in the google search bar. Using social media can be a great way for you to reach out to other people who are going through the same experiences that you have. It is good to find other outlets that can be just as helpful as your family especially as you are becoming an adult. There will be times that you are not at home like if you go off to college, spend a night at your friends or take a vacation these times you will be alone no mom around and it will be up to you to remember how to handle your own care.

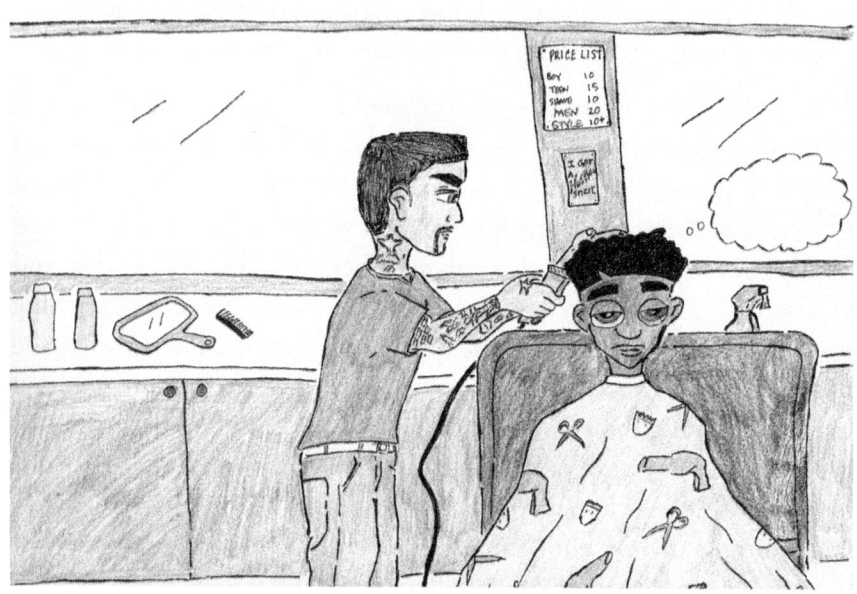

It had been about a year since the stroke things had gone back to normal for the most part everyone fell back into their routines and for a while things were normal. Lee had lost interest in all his hobbies, school was another challenge he had to face. Getting back into school was intimidating in some ways because he would be older so he decided to enroll in a school online which was very helpful because of his age he decided that he wanted to take his G.E.D

Surviving against the odds is something that Lee had done he knew that by the age twenty only 20% of sickle cell children beat the odds of having a stroke. Leaving 80% who have another stroke occurrence within three years of the first. It is a possibility that the child may have little strokes that can affect how your child thinks, function or even alter parts of their personality. Having transfusions done every four weeks is a strategical move by the hematology team to keep the hemoglobin S level below 30% to detour another stroke from occurring. Once transfusions start monthly you are not supposed to stop them this could cause another stroke as well.

Lee often thought of what he wanted to do in life he made a decision to live without fear of the unknown. Seeing how quickly life could change he wanted to tell others about having sickle cell because it seemed like when he would talk about it very few knew what it was. Knowing that he would always have to get a transfusion to stop from having a stroke made him think about the blood supply and what if they ran out and what could he do to help the sickle cell community. Noticing that he would think about ways he could contribute to his own illness gave him control over his illness in his eyes.

Now that Angel has been gone with dad over a year it was just Minnie and Lee which at times was lonely for him. Brothers have a bond that is unbreakable the miles between them is the only thing that keeps them from hanging out like they used to. The time that has passed left Lee thinking what he would do after graduating and how he had to start paying attention to all the things his mom has been telling him so he can learn how to manage his own care. Hard stuff to admit is when you have not been applying yourself with your fullest capabilities. His mom had been on him to start making his own appointments and scheduling transportation pickups that his insurance provides for free.

Drawn into the kitchen by the smell of fish frying Lee found his mom in front of the stove cooking dinner. He came in saying "You know I can fry fish that better than you mom?!" She turned around smiling as she saw Lee walking towards her with his arms out to get a quick hug, she giggled "Hey there, what are you up too? How was your day baby?" Lee replied saying "It was fine but I wanted to talk to you about the things you have done to take care of my sickle cell. I know I am older now so I am ready to learn how to handle my own care."

Lee sat down with his mom and told her about his plan to pursue music production, art and culinary school. She always encouraged him to use his natural talents of drawing because she too was an artist. His mother always told her children to embrace their talents, learn a skill, be passionate about their trade and always include their dreams in their goals. When Lee was in occupational therapy he was able to reignite his skills in the kitchen laughing his mom could see his eyes light up as he talks about cooking again what drawing has him thinking of art as a form of therapy. Those jobs that are not physically demanding and won't compromise your health are ideal for someone with sickle cell.

Music is a universal tool that touches everything is comes in contact with all of art are forms of expression and communication which Lee had to learn all over again. The hematology team and the arts brought him back to life so as his mom she thought

"I will give him these tools to go out into the world". His family all grew up listening to hip hop from the 80s and 90s, his mom would clean the house to singing her favorite Aaliyah, Ashanti or Mary J. Blige song. She encouraged all of her children being a young mom she was very close to them not only did she raise them she grew up with them as well. They became her reason to be a better person and overcome what obstacles despite the doubt on all levels in her life she did just that.

She thought about the day when he would be ready voluntarily to handle his own care and all of the days she spent making sure he was at every appointment is now primarily his responsibility. As a mother we all know that we will never just stop being a mother but there are times when you have to stop telling your child who has grown into an adult what to do. Giving your child suggestions with different options like a multiple choice is the best way for them to choose and you plant the seed of different scenarios in their own mind.

For the last nineteen years she had protected him it was time for him to see a few things on his own knowing she will have his back meant the most to Lee. Asking around he found out there are so many myths about sickle cell that had to be clarified and one of the biggest is that only black or African decent have the traits and this is wrong. Many backgrounds with different ethnicities such as Italian, Arabian, Greek, Turkish, Israeli, Pakistani, and Latin so all newborns should be screened at birth. Many cultures have blended in the last fifty years knowing your genetic background and sharing that with who you are having a relationship will be the best way to prevent the unknown possibility of carrying a trait that could harm your child's future family.

The best advice is if you are not sure ask your doctor, look it up on a trusted website, get a book and read but do your research. Get involved in mentoring a younger child with sickle cell, volunteer in the same hospital that you were at during pain crisis as a child. All of this will help with your own struggles by being able to pass on knowledge and experience that you have lived through it will give them courage and fill some of the spaces in life sickle cell has filled in a not so pleasant way. Getting involved in your place of worship will keep you grounded and provide a huge place for inspiration and comfort.

One of the big challenges will be how to manage the pain growing up Lee mastered some basic skills like the hot bath, massage if needed his mom would work up to his pain medication depending on his pain level. Keeping a record of the pain and its location can be very helpful all should be in a pain log.

PAIN LOG

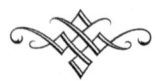

PAIN LOG

DATE/TIME						
LOCATION						
PAIN LEVEL						
TYPE OF PAIN						
SYMPTOMS						
ENVIRONMENT						

KEEPING TRACK

Documenting the details and giving description can be key to finding the triggers for a pain crisis. If the pain is dull, throbbing, sharp, burning for example would give direction on how to treat the pain quickly. Once you are in pain know how to handle it and remember to treat it according to the level of pain. If your pain is severe and accompanied by a fever of 101 degrees you must get to the emergency room. If you are able to handle it at home you might want to try the heat compress, soaking, meditation and then take medication if pain progresses. Understand your proper dosage and combinations of medication trying all of these methods should get you through the pain episode. If you are doing all of your home methods with no success or you are having the red flag symptoms of a fever, headache, chest pain, abdominal pain you must go to the emergency room.

Often the pain is difficult so you would want to try all the pain techniques you know so using the stronger pain medication is your only choice. Having sickle cell anemia Lee has managed his pain all his life with the help of his mother he didn't have to worry about using medication too often although he did have a higher tolerance for pain than most. To avoid developing a physical dependence on the medication that had opiates in it Lee limited his use of those. Becoming an adult with sickle cell who deals with pain that will come and go forever it is important to educate them on drug abuse to prevent the use for depression and pain control.

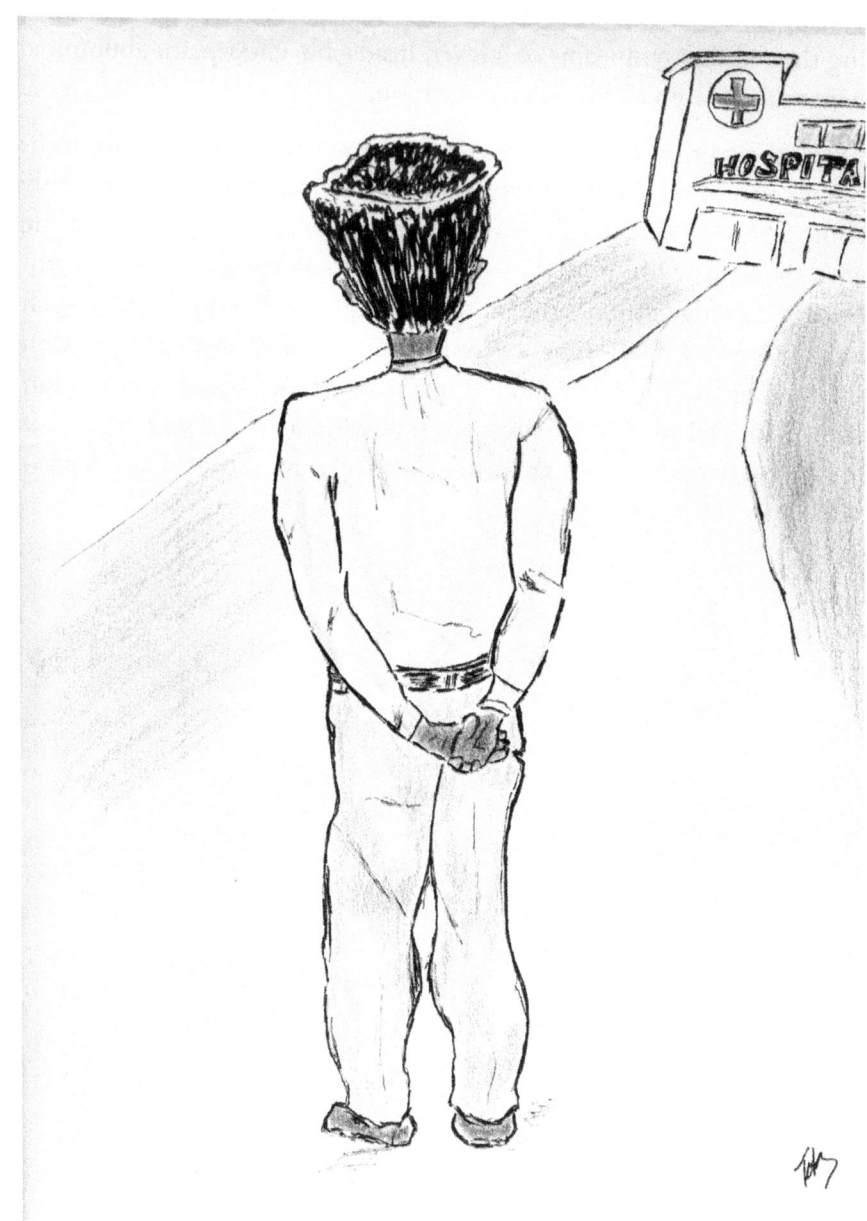

Living independently is any young adult's goal who is motivated to get out on their own. Keeping all your appointments will be up to you for the most part you will have to schedule the appointments, transportation to and from, and keep records of any issues. Missing appointments can lead to you being undertreated leaving you unable to handle your pain with limited medication and outdated prescriptions this would lead to searching for alternative methods to handle pain some that can be harmful and mislabel you as a drug addict.

Meditation, relaxing techniques will save you from dwelling on how bad the pain feels. Yoga can take you to a calm peaceful place as you work your muscles and get through the pain. Going to your medical team to come up with your independent pain management plan is a proactive way to handle your care.

Armed with knowledge of how to take care of his illness Lee was able to confidently start his next phase in life with sickle cell anemia. Looking at him most see a young black man with his hip hop swag, ear phones in his ears, bobbing his head to his music. With his hat pulled down low framing his not so yellow eyes (getting transfusions keeps his eyes clearer) Lee always assumed he had nothing more threatening in his life then the streets in his neighborhood. He realized that years ago the medical community said that life expectancy is going up with all of the adequate prevention, modern treatments, education information, genetic counseling and good health care combined with healthy living. Being prepared a person with sickle cell can have a family, become a lawyer, computer technician or artist contributing to your communities and sickle cell anemia awareness and research.

THE END

HEALTH PASSPORT

MEDICAL INFORMATION TO KEEP

NAME: _____

DATE OF BIRTH: _____

SICKLE CELL TYPE (SBth, SC,SS): _____

DOCTOR: _____

DR. PHONE #: __(_____)_____-_____-_____

HOSPITAL: _____

MEDICAL RECORD #: _____

ALLERGIES: _____

MEDICATION: _____

_____

PAIN MEDICATIONS: _____

ER PAIN MEDICATIONS: _____

PHARMACY: _____

PHONE: _____(_____)_____-_____-_____

COMPLICATIONS: _____

_____

_____

TRANSFUSIONS: _____

SURGERIES: _____

RESOURCES

www.stjude.org for St. Jude research hospital

www.hematology.org for the American society of hematology

www.scinfo.org for medical providers online 24 hours a day

www.stroke.org for current information on stroke awareness.

www.sicklecelldisease.org for the sickle cell disease association of America.

www.ascaa.org for the American sickle cell anemia association

www.sicklecellsociety.org for the sickle cell society of London, England

www.ampainsoc.org for the American pain society

DO YOUR HOMEWORK!

YouTube has free videos and an online community be sure to type "sickle cell" in the search bar. Just about everyone has a profile on one of the social media platforms like Facebook, Instagram, or Twitter and if you type in sickle cell on the search bar countless people, groups, foundations related to sickle cell. Technology has been a bridge when it comes to providing information, doing research, and connecting people all over the world from all walks of life.

#SICKLECELLKIDD @SICKLECELLKIDD

DEDICATION

This book is written in loving memory of Clarice Shepherd my grand-mother who was the foundation and heart of my family. I dedicate it to anyone who has or had a loved one with sickle cell anemia and all who ever dreamed of being an artist and writer.

A portion of the proceeds of this book will help bring awareness, and research for Sickle Cell Awareness and Advocacy. A percentage will help fund #sicklecellkidd education and supporter projects.